Shedding Pounds, Finding Freedom

A Comprehensive Guide book to Overcoming Obesity

By

Dr Angela D. Smith

Table of content

DISCLAIMER

The material contained in this book, titled "Shedding Pounds, Finding Freedom," serves merely as general informational assistance and should not be taken as a replacement for professional medical advice, diagnosis, or treatment. The author and publisher of this book are not medical experts, and the material contained herein should not be construed as medical advice.

The contents of this book are anchored on the author's research, personal experiences, and knowledge acquired from credible sources. However, individual situations fluctuate, and the information may not be appropriate for everyone. It is highly advised that readers get counsel and direction from certified healthcare specialists about their unique health ailments or concerns.

Every attempt has been made to guarantee the accuracy and timeliness of the material contained in this book. Nonetheless, the approaches, ideas, and advice presented cannot guarantee precise outcomes for every person. Outcomes may vary depending on variables such as individual health problems, genetics, lifestyle choices, and adherence to the advice stated. Readers are asked to utilize their judgment and caution while adopting any advice from this book.

The author and publisher do not support any specific diet, fitness regimen, or product featured in this book. Any suggestions made are merely for informative reasons and should not be taken as endorsements. Readers are recommended to perform their research and speak with healthcare specialists before making any changes to their diet, exercise regimen, or lifestyle.

By buying and reading this book, you acknowledge your understanding and consent to the conditions described in the Disclaimer. Thank you for joining us on this exciting adventure.

Printed in [United States of America].
Published by [Admus Groups Printing Limited].
For permissions, please contact [admusgruopprintinglimited@gmail.com]

PART 1 INTRODUCTION

Obesity is a serious public health problem that affects millions of people worldwide. Because of its rising prevalence and severe impact on physical, emotional, and mental health, it is frequently referred to as an epidemic. Obesity not only enhances the risk of chronic diseases such as heart disease, stroke, diabetes, and cancer, but it may also have a devastating influence on a person's social and economic situation. Despite diverse initiatives to address the problem, its prevalence continues to increase, underscoring the need for a more comprehensive approach to obesity prevention. This is where this book comes in: it offers a fresh and creative approach to battling obesity by emphasizing several areas that contribute to the illness. The book delivers readers practical tools, expert counsel, and effective strategies to help them lose weight and improve their overall health. Whether you're battling with obesity or simply attempting to maintain a healthy weight, this book is a valuable resource that will help you take responsibility for your health and change your life for the better.

CHAPTER 1

WHAT EXACTLY IS OBESITY?

Obesity is a difficult medical illness characterized by an unusually high amount of body fat. Obesity is defined by the World Health Organization (WHO) as having a body mass index (BMI) of 30 or more. The body mass index (BMI) is a measurement of weight. based on height and weight.

Obesity is caused by a combination of inherited, environmental, and behavioral factors. Obesity susceptibility is influenced by genetic predisposition. Access to bad food alternatives, a lack of physical activity, and sedentary lifestyles may all contribute to weight gain. Weight growth may also be impacted by behavioral factors such as eating habits, stress, and a lack of sleep.

When people consume more calories than their bodies burn, the surplus calories are stored as fat.

This additional fat accumulates over time, leading to weight rise. The probability of having obesity-related health disorders grows as weight rises.

Obesity is connected with many major health concerns. Obese persons are more prone to get type 2 diabetes, high blood pressure, heart disease, stroke, sleep apnea, and several kinds of cancer. Obesity may also contribute to the development of mental health issues such as melancholy, worry, and low self-esteem. These health dangers may ultimately result in a shorter lifespan, a lower quality of life, and greater healthcare expenses.

Obesity is a condition caused by a combination of genetic, environmental, and behavioral factors. It is characterized by an abnormal increase in body fat and is related to numerous significant health concerns. Treatment and prevention methods include dietary adjustments and, in some instances, pharmaceutical therapies.

I. Age, gender, and ethnicity are all variables that contribute to obesity.

People's metabolisms slow down as they age, and they lose muscle mass, making it easier to gain weight. Women store more fat than males, especially in the hips and thighs, which may contribute to weight gain and obesity. Obesity and accompanying health conditions are more widespread in particular ethnic groups, such as African Americans, Hispanics, and Native Americans.

Obesity has a deleterious effect on both individual and public health. Obesity is a worldwide concern that is a leading cause of unnecessary death and disability. Obesity has a considerable economic effect owing to greater healthcare expenses and lost productivity. As a consequence, fighting the obesity epidemic is a public health priority.

While obesity is a multifaceted illness caused by a multitude of situations, the public health effects of obesity are immense. To combat the obesity epidemic, a multimodal approach that encompasses human behavior change as well as legislative and environmental measures is necessary.

Understanding Obesity

Yes, understanding obesity may be hard and requires a full explanation owing to the various variables involved. To begin, obesity is a medical illness in which a person's body fat exceeds a reasonable range, resulting in serious health implications. Obesity is assessed using the Body Mass Index (BMI), and a BMI of 30 or above denotes obesity.

Lifestyle choices, particularly overeating and a lack of physical activity, are primary reasons for obesity. Consuming high-calorie meals, especially ones rich in sugar and fat, may contribute to weight gain, and if this practice is sustained, it may lead to obesity. A sedentary lifestyle, in which individuals do not engage in regular physical activity, such as exercise, also contributes to weight increase and obesity.

Other characteristics that contribute to obesity include genetic susceptibility, underlying medical problems such as hypothyroidism, stress, socioeconomic level, and poor sleep.

Some individuals, for example, have a hereditary inclination to accumulate weight, making it easy for them to grow obese. Chronic stress may elevate cortisol levels in the body, which may lead to weight gain. Sleep deprivation may also affect hormones that control appetite, leading to increased urges for high-calorie meals.

Furthermore, obesity is connected with a variety of health concerns. It boosts the probability of obtaining chronic diseases such as type 2 diabetes, hypertension, heart disease, stroke, some cancers, sleep apnea, and osteoarthritis. Obesity may also have a detrimental influence on mental health, leading to low self-esteem, melancholy, anxiety, and social bias.

<u>There are two forms of bodily fat</u>

It is necessary to analyze the different kinds of body fat. Visceral fat and subcutaneous fat are the two kinds of body fat. Visceral fat is a kind of fat that surrounds the organs and may induce insulin resistance, high blood pressure, and dyslipidemia. Subcutaneous fat, on the other hand, is positioned directly beneath the skin and may be seen and pressed. While subcutaneous fat is less harmful than visceral fat, it may still create health risks in large amounts.

People of all ages, genders, and socioeconomic backgrounds are impacted by obesity. Certain populations, however, are more prone to obesity than others. People living in low-income regions, for example, may have limited access to nutritional meals and safe venues to exercise, increasing their risk of obesity. Furthermore, in many cultures, overweight individuals are considered healthy and attractive, which may lead to a lack of desire to engage in physical activity and maintain a healthy weight.

It is vital to remember that obesity is a chronic illness that requires long-term management. Fad diets or rapid fixes are useless in the long term and may be detrimental to one's health. Individuals should instead undertake long-term lifestyle improvements such as including more fruits and vegetables in their meals, limiting portion sizes, and increasing physical activity. Regular physical activity and exercise may also promote overall physical and mental health and minimize the risk of chronic diseases.

It should be mentioned that knowing obesity requires an examination of the different variables and events that contribute to it. Obesity's diverse nature needs a comprehensive approach to adequately addressing the disease. Individuals may lessen their risk of obesity and increase their overall well-being by enhancing general health and making sustainable lifestyle modifications.

Body Mass Index (BMI)

Body Mass Index (BMI) is a frequently used clinical measure for measuring an individual's weight status and the associated health concerns related to their weight. BMI is a measure of body weight in proportion to height that is produced by dividing an individual's weight in kilograms by their height in meters squared (kg/m2). BMI is a common measurement as it is quick to obtain and non-invasive, making it a helpful tool for healthcare practitioners.

BMI is used to define weight status into four traditional categories: underweight, healthy weight, overweight, and obese. A BMI of less than 18.5 is considered underweight, but a BMI of 18.5 to 24.9 is considered healthy weight. A BMI of 25 to 29.9 is considered obese,

while obesity is defined as a BMI of 30 or higher. Higher BMI levels are related to higher risks of a range of health concerns, including cardiovascular disease, diabetes, musculoskeletal diseases, and numerous cancers.

While BMI is an important tool, it is not without constraints. BMI, for example, does not discriminate between fat mass and lean mass, which can lead to an overestimation of obesity in people with a lot of muscle mass. Furthermore, BMI does not account for differences in body composition among ethnicities, which may result in varying health risks for persons of diverse races and ethnic backgrounds. Furthermore, BMI may not adequately reflect results in pregnant or lactating women, athletes, and the elderly, as their body composition and metabolism differ from those of healthy persons.

BMI is typically used by physicians in combination with other health metrics, such as waist circumference, blood pressure, cholesterol levels, and glucose tolerance, to appropriately estimate an individual's overall health risk. This allows therapists to build a personalized approach to weight management, lifestyle therapies, and medications for health optimization and weight-related disease management. Using BMI and other clinical indicators, healthcare practitioners may give individualized health recommendations to patients and boost health outcomes, all while preventing and controlling present and future obesity and related chronic disease epidemics.

BMI may be used to assess the progress of weight reduction endeavors in addition to accurately examining an individual's weight status and health issues. Individuals who are urged to lose weight and have a high BMI could use BMI as a tool to develop weight reduction goals and assess their success over time. This could help individuals stay motivated and on track with their weight loss aims.

While BMI is not a perfect metric for gauging weight and health risks, it remains a common clinical tool due to its simplicity, practicality, and ability to present a rapid assessment of an individual's complete weight status. However, healthcare practitioners must remember that BMI is only one component of a comprehensive examination of an individual's health and should not be used to make treatment recommendations on its own.

By combining BMI with other health measurements and clinical assessments, healthcare practitioners may present patients with tailored health recommendations and increase health outcomes. However, BMI should be understood in the context of a person's circumstances and risk factors, since this will allow for more effective and customized health management.

CHAPTER 2

OBESITY IN DIFFERENT AGE GROUPS

Obesity is a serious public health concern that affects persons of all ages, including children and the elderly. It is described as having a BMI of 30 or more, suggesting additional body fat and a heightened risk of a variety of health concerns.

Obesity is a serious issue in adolescents, as it may lead to a range of health difficulties such as diabetes, hypertension, sleep apnea, and even early death in adulthood if not treated. Children who are overweight or obese are also more likely to be bullied and endure social stigma, which may impair their mental health and self-esteem.

Obesity poses severe health concerns in youngsters as well. Diabetes, hypertension, cardiovascular disease, joint issues, and perhaps cancer are all heightened risks. Furthermore, studies have shown that obese teens are more prone to develop depression and anxiety, underlining the importance of early intervention and prevention.

Obesity may lead to a variety of health issues in young and middle-aged persons, including diabetes, cardiovascular disease, hypertension, sleep apnea, and various kinds of cancer. It may also reduce life expectancy and quality of life, exerting pressure on healthcare institutions and society as a whole.

Obesity may have a considerable effect on physical function and mobility in older adults. It elevates the probability of falls and fractures, resulting in diminished independence and increased healthcare expenses. It also raises the risk of various age-related health concerns like heart disease, stroke, and cognitive decline.

It should be mentioned that the effect of obesity on health differs depending on individual conditions such as underlying health concerns, genetics, and lifestyle factors. Furthermore, treatment and management of obesity may change depending on age and other clinical concerns.

Obesity affects persons of all ages, and its influence on health varies according to age and other clinical problems. Prevention and early intervention are crucial in minimizing the health hazards associated with obesity, and healthcare practitioners should investigate individualized treatment and management strategies based on an individual's particular circumstances.

Obesity has enormous economic repercussions in addition to the health difficulties it causes. Obesity-related healthcare expenses may strain healthcare systems and lead to greater healthcare spending. Obesity's economic toll may include missed productivity due to absenteeism and poorer job competence, as well as greater costs linked with disability and early mortality.

Furthermore, the impact of obesity on health is not isolated to the individual but may have a cascade effect on their families and communities. Obesity, for example, can elevate the risk of related health issues in family members and impose extra stress on caretakers.

Prevention and intervention strategies that target multiple factors, such as lifestyle adjustments, social support, and policy changes, may be useful in decreasing obesity prevalence across all age groups. Promoting good eating habits, physical activity, and regular weight monitoring in adolescents may assist to prevent and treat obesity before it becomes a severe health concern.

Interventions concentrating on weight reduction and management, as well as the prevention and treatment of related health conditions, may serve to increase quality of life and minimize healthcare expenses in middle-aged and older adults. In some instances, these interventions may entail lifestyle adjustments, pharmacological control, and surgical procedures.

Obesity is a significant public health issue that affects individuals of all ages and has major health and economic repercussions. To properly address the impacts of obesity on health and well-being, a comprehensive and customized approach to prevention and treatment is necessary.

Obesity Factors

Obesity is a multifaceted condition caused by a combination of genetic, environmental, and behavioral factors. The primary causes of obesity are categorized into various groups in a therapeutic setting.

Genetics: A person's genes may have a major role in obesity development. Certain genes, according to studies, may impact a person's metabolism, hormone management, and the way fat is stored in the body. People with a family history of obesity are more prone to get the illness themselves.

Environmental factors such as diet, physical activity levels, and sleep patterns may all have a part in the development of obesity. A diet high in calories, saturated fats, and sweets may result in weight gain over time. Obesity may also be caused by a lack of physical activity, which restricts the body from burning enough calories to maintain a healthy weight. Sleep deprivation may impair the body's metabolic functions, which may lead to obesity.

Behavioral factors: Stress, pharmacological side effects, and smoking may all contribute to the development of obesity. Stress may change appetite and lead to overeating. Weight gain may be an adverse effect of several medicines, such as antidepressants. Smoking may also contribute to obesity by changing metabolism and promoting weight gain.

Medical conditions: Obesity may also be caused by certain medical disorders. Hormone imbalances such as hypothyroidism, Cushing's disease, and polycystic ovarian syndrome (PCOS) are examples. Obesity may also be caused by various medical conditions such as Prader-Willi syndrome, genetic disorders, and hypothalamic lesions.

Despite its complexity, obesity is an illness that, with the right therapy, may be effectively treated and managed. To aid patients in attaining and keeping a healthy weight, healthcare specialists typically suggest a combination of dietary adjustment, physical activity, behavioral therapy, and medication.

Diet modification comprises making alterations to one's diet to lower calorie intake and increase nutritional balance. This can mean eating more fruits and vegetables, choosing lean protein sources, decreasing portion sizes, and avoiding meals heavy in fat, sugar, and salt.

Physical activity is also a vital aspect of treating obesity. To help patients burn calories and increase general wellness, healthcare practitioners frequently suggest at least 150 minutes of moderate-intensity exercise each week. Exercise could vary from brisk walking to jogging, cycling, and swimming.

Patients could benefit from behavioral therapy to address the psychological and emotional factors that contribute to overeating and weight gain. This may incorporate cognitive behavioral therapy, mindfulness-based stress reduction, and other stress-reduction treatments.

In rare cases, healthcare practitioners may also encourage patients to utilize medication to aid them in losing weight. Appetite suppressants, which may help lessen food cravings and support weight loss, as well as medications that target certain metabolic pathways that contribute to obesity, are examples of pharmaceuticals.

Bariatric surgery may be indicated for those who are severely obese and have not been able to achieve acceptable weight loss through other treatments. The surgical alteration of the digestive system to reduce the amount of food a person may ingest or the number of calories absorbed from meals is known as bariatric surgery.

Finally, the most effective technique for obesity therapy is one that treats all of the condition's underlying causes. Patients may accomplish large and sustained weight loss by cooperating with healthcare practitioners to build a personalized treatment strategy that includes dietary modification, physical activity, behavioral counseling, and medication (if necessary).

The Obesity Epidemic

The obesity pandemic refers to the recent large and widespread increase in the prevalence of obesity in the general population. The term "epidemic" is used as the prevalence of obesity has swiftly grown and impacted a significant number of persons, making it a serious public health concern.

Obesity has a huge and well-documented effect on health. It has been connected to several chronic illnesses such as type 2 diabetes, cardiovascular disease, certain cancers, and mental health concerns. These diseases may place a substantial load on the healthcare system while also leading to early mortality and a lower quality of life for people who suffer from them.

Clinically, the obesity epidemic demands a multifaceted management plan combining healthcare practitioners, governments, and individuals. This may include community-based programs that encourage access to nutritional meals and safe venues for physical exercise, as well as interventions that promote healthy lifestyle choices such as regular physical activity and a balanced diet. Furthermore, healthcare specialists may administer counseling, behavioral therapy, and medication to aid patients in obtaining and maintaining a healthy weight. Finally, preventing and controlling obesity involves a systematic and continuing effort that targets the myriad elements that contribute to this condition.

The obesity epidemic has become a worldwide concern, with an estimated 650 million obese persons globally. According to the Centers for Disease Control and Prevention (CDC), the United States has the biggest proportion of obese persons, at roughly 36.5%. Childhood obesity is also on the increase, with roughly 18% of children aged 6 to 11 and 21% of children aged 12 to 19 categorized as obese.

The causes of the obesity epidemic are diverse and complex. They include genetic susceptibility as well as environmental factors such as high-energy meals, sedentary lifestyles, sleep deprivation, and stress. The accessible availability of high-calorie foods and beverages, coupled with a lack of physical exercise, means that many individuals consume more calories than they burn over lengthy periods.

The obesity epidemic has had a major impact, with considerable health repercussions.

Obesity is associated with a range of medical concerns that may lead to disability and even death. Heart disease, stroke, diabetes, osteoarthritis, certain cancers, sleep apnea, and chronic kidney illness are examples. Other health dangers connected with these illnesses include hypertension, dyslipidemia, insulin resistance, and inflammation.

Obesity prevention and control necessitate a multimodal public health approach that tackles linked challenges at the individual, organizational, and community levels. Promoting healthy and active lives, such as good eating and regular exercise, reducing sedentary habits, providing access to nutritional foods, and creating settings that foster healthy lifestyles are all techniques for avoiding and controlling obesity.

 The obesity epidemic offers a tremendous public health risk. Effective obesity prevention and control require long-term multimodal solutions at the individual, organizational, and community levels. To address the complex and diverse factors creating the obesity epidemic, healthcare professionals, lawmakers, and communities will need to work together.

CHAPTER 3

OBESITY CONSEQUENCES

Obesity boosts the probability of getting many medical illnesses and may exacerbate pre-existing ones. Type 2 diabetes, hypertension, hyperlipidemia, coronary artery disease, heart failure, stroke, sleep apnea, fatty liver disease, osteoarthritis, and various kinds of cancer are examples of such disorders. Obesity boosts the chance of insulin resistance, which may evolve into type 2 diabetes. Excess body fat puts pressure on the heart, leading to hypertension and heart disease.

Obesity also generates inflammation in the body, which may lead to chronic, low-grade inflammation, which may contribute to the development of a variety of various ailments. It may also create respiratory concerns, such as asthma, and make it difficult to participate in physical exercise, which may lead to a sedentary lifestyle, worsening the illness.

Obesity may induce social isolation, sorrow, poor self-esteem, and a terrible quality of life. Obese persons may face prejudice and discrimination, resulting in social stigmatization, which may compound these psychological repercussions. These effects may create a vicious cycle in which obese persons turn to food as a coping technique, leading to even greater weight gain.

Obesity may also have a financial consequence. Obese persons may have fewer career opportunities, inferior income, and greater healthcare costs as a consequence of the underlying medical conditions. Obesity's economic toll extends beyond the individual to society as a whole, exerting huge financial pressure on healthcare systems.

Obesity may be caused by a combination of genetic factors, eating choices, and lifestyle habits. The underlying causes of obesity, however, are varied and diverse, making therapy challenging. The most effective obesity treatment is weight reduction by lifestyle adjustments such as a balanced diet and regular exercise. For patients who are exceedingly obese, several medicines and weight reduction techniques may be tried.

The key to decreasing the health consequences of obesity is prevention. Obesity may be prevented by developing excellent food and physical activity habits, limiting sedentary behavior, and cultivating a healthy lifestyle from an early age. Government rules, such as charges on unhealthy foods and encouragement for physical activity, may also help to a healthier lifestyle.

Obesity has various consequences that have a considerable influence on one's health, both physically and emotionally. To minimize the negative health implications of obesity, it is necessary to treat it with lifestyle adjustments such as exercise, a decent diet, stress management, quality sleep, and smoking cessation, among other strategies.

Obesity's Health Risks

Obesity has been associated with a variety of health concerns and is considered a serious public health issue. Obesity-related extra body fat development may have a range of clinical consequences on various biological systems.

Cardiovascular disease is one of the most frequently acknowledged health dangers with obesity. Obesity enhances the risk of hypertension, dyslipidemia, and atherosclerosis, all of which contribute to the start of heart disease such as coronary artery disease, myocardial infarction, and stroke.

Obesity is also connected to an increased risk of type 2 diabetes. Excess body fat impairs the insulin response, leading to insulin resistance and the development of type 2 diabetes. Obese persons are two to four times more likely to get type 2 diabetes than healthy-weight people.

Obesity elevates the risk of numerous kinds of cancer, including colorectal, breast, and endometrial cancer, in addition to cardiovascular disease and type 2 diabetes. Cancer is thought to be induced by inflammation, hormonal imbalances, and changes in insulin resistance caused by obesity.

Obesity also elevates the risk of a variety of other medical conditions, including sleep apnea, nonalcoholic fatty liver disease, osteoarthritis, gout, and chronic kidney illness. These conditions have the potential to cause severe morbidity and mortality.

Obesity may also produce musculoskeletal difficulties due to increased joint pressure. This may lead to conditions like arthritis and continuous discomfort, making it difficult for individuals to go about their usual routines.

Obesity has also been associated with respiratory disorders like asthma and sleep apnea. The additional weight may put pressure on the lungs, making breathing harder and boosting the risk of respiratory illnesses.

Obesity is also connected to mental health difficulties like unhappiness, worry, and low self-esteem. Obesity's social stigma may lead to discrimination, shame, and isolation, leading to additional mental health concerns in individuals.

It is vital to note that the health concerns related to obesity differ depending on where the body fat accumulates. Individuals with higher abdominal fat are more prone to develop heart disease and type 2 diabetes than those with more fat accumulation in their hips and thighs.

Obesity is preventable and manageable with a healthy lifestyle that includes regular exercise and a well-balanced diet. Maintaining a healthy weight minimizes the probability of having obesity-related chronic health conditions. When lifestyle adjustments are inadequate to treat obesity, medical procedures such as bariatric surgery may be investigated.

Obesity is a difficult medical disorder that brings a lot of health dangers. To prevent and cure obesity, it is vital to improve understanding of the condition and its linked health dangers. Adopting healthy lifestyle improvements, such as regular exercise and a well-balanced diet, is crucial for living a healthier life.

Obesity's Effect on Mental Health

Obesity is a difficult health condition that may affect both an individual's physical and mental well-being. Obesity's impact on mental health is thoroughly documented and may appear in several ways. Obesity's social stigma may lead to prejudice and prejudgment of persons with the condition, which may result in negative psychological repercussions such as despair and anxiety. Labeling obesity as a personal or lifestyle choice rather than a medical diagnosis may compound the issue and lead to a lack of community understanding and assistance.

Obesity may also have a significant effect on a person's self-esteem and body image, resulting in negative thoughts and feelings of shame and self-doubt. Obesity is related to a lack of self-control and moral failure, which adds to emotions of shame and internalized stigma. These characteristics lead to poor self-perception, which may impair an individual's ability to participate socially, resulting in undesirable mental health outcomes such as social isolation and loneliness.

Obesity may also produce neuroendocrine abnormalities, changing brain function and behavior and leading to mood disorders like depression. Adipose tissue, or fat, is an active endocrine organ that creates hormones such as leptin, adiponectin, and ghrelin. Leptin and adiponectin are hormones that influence hunger, energy expenditure, insulin sensitivity, and glucose metabolism. Ghrelin, on the other hand, is responsible for signaling hunger and fullness.

Obese persons have altered hormone production, resulting in chronic inflammation and hormonal imbalances that may contribute to the development of mood disorders.

Obesity-related hormonal imbalances may affect brain function, resulting in anatomical abnormalities and cognitive impairment. It may also affect memory, attention, and decision-making skills, leading to poor academic or vocational performance.

Obesity may create sentiments of guilt, sorrow, and despair, limiting a person's capacity to interact socially and accomplish routine duties. Obesity-related neuroendocrine abnormalities may affect brain function and lead to mood disorders such as depression and cognitive impairment. It is vital to address the effect of obesity on mental health to increase the overall well-being of persons suffering from the condition.

Obesity may also induce sleep issues such as sleep apnea, which may exacerbate its effect on mental health. Sleep apnea is a condition in which breathing repeatedly pauses and restarts during sleep, resulting in sleep disturbance and fatigue throughout the day. A higher risk of depression, anxiety, and other mood disorders has been associated with this condition. It may also induce cognitive impairment and poor attention, both of which may impede a person's overall functioning.

Obesity has been connected to the development of stress-related disorders. Chronic stress from living with obesity, together with societal stigma, may lead to the development of stress-related illnesses such as post-traumatic stress disorder (PTSD), anxiety disorders, and obsessive-compulsive disorder (OCD). Obesity-related sentiments of guilt and shame may also trigger the development of chronic illnesses, resulting in a decline in overall quality of life.

Obesity may also have a harmful influence on one's quality of life by lowering one's ability to engage in physical activities, which may lead to higher social isolation and unpleasant mood symptoms. Inactivity may also contribute to the development of stress-related disorders and cognitive impairment.

Obesity's effect on mental health must be addressed by a multidisciplinary approach that involves healthcare practitioners, mental health professionals, and community assistance. The medical profession should embrace a more holistic approach to obesity treatment, incorporating both physical and mental health results. Individuals with obesity may benefit from the aid of mental health professionals in dealing with the emotional and social challenges that come with the condition, which may enhance overall well-being.

Obesity may have a big effect on mental health via a range of physiological and psychological reasons. The frequency of mood and stress-related disorders is enhanced by social stigma, poor self-perception, cognitive degradation, sleep problems, and a reduced quality of life. To promote the well-being of persons suffering from obesity, complete treatment is essential, including treating mental health concerns.

<u>Obstacles to Living with Obesity</u>

One of the major difficulties of living with obesity is cultural stigma.

Discrimination and prejudice may result in negative self-perception, feelings of shame, and low self-esteem. These emotional responses may create psychological suffering and lead to worry, depression, and other mood disorders.

Chronic stress is also a huge concern for persons who are obese, as they may encounter ongoing societal demands and persistent weight management difficulties, both of which may contribute to chronic stress. Stress-related diseases such as post-traumatic stress disorder (PTSD), generalized anxiety disorder (GAD), obsessive-compulsive disorder (OCD), and other mood disorders may develop as a consequence of continuous stress.

Furthermore, obesity-related difficulties such as decreased physical activity and mobility may lead to feelings of social isolation, depression, and worry. These limits may aggravate the issues associated with obesity by reducing an individual's ability to engage in physical activities and social connections, both of which are crucial for general well-being and mental health.

Obesity is also connected to a host of disorders that could hurt a person's mental health. Social stigma, sleep problems, chronic stress, social isolation, and limited mobility are all elements that could lead to emotional discomfort and mood disorders. To treat both the physical and emotional health implications of obesity, healthcare providers, mental health experts, and community support must take a holistic approach to therapy.

The problems of living with obesity extend beyond the person and could affect the individual's family and social support network. Family members may feel helpless or frustrated in their attempts to support their loved one in controlling their weight, resulting in strained relationships and added stress in the family. Individuals with obesity may endure discrimination or stigmatization from friends and acquaintances, leading to feelings of isolation and lower social support, which may influence social support networks.

Emotional eating and body image disorders are two psychological components that could contribute to the challenges of living with obesity. Emotional eating is caused by stress, anxiety, or sadness. response that may lead to overeating and weight gain, perpetuating the obesity cycle. Body image difficulties may also contribute to poor self-perception and low self-esteem, exacerbating emotional discomfort. Obesity poses several hurdles, including social stigma, health problems, disruptions in family and social support, psychological concerns, and lower quality of life. As a result, a thorough treatment plan is crucial in addressing the physical and mental health effects of this illness.

PART 2 DIET AND EXERCISE

Diet and exercise" is a typical phrase used to symbolize two significant lifestyle adjustments that may aid individuals in obtaining and maintaining a healthy weight.

Eating a balanced diet that includes selections from all food categories (fruits, vegetables, grains, protein, dairy, fats) and limiting consumption of foods rich in calories, sugar, and saturated fats may help people reach and maintain a healthy weight.

Regular exercise, such as walking, running, swimming, cycling, or weightlifting, can help individuals achieve a healthy weight by burning excess calories. Exercise can also benefit overall physical and mental health by improving cardiovascular health, reducing inflammation in the body, improving mood, and reducing stress.

To achieve long-term success in weight control, it is vital to find a balance between diet and exercise; neither can work successfully on its own.

A healthy diet helps to limit calorie intake while also providing the body with the nutrients it requires for optimal health. Incorporating whole, nutrient-dense foods like fruits, vegetables, and lean protein sources like fish, chicken, and beans can keep hunger at bay while also providing the body with the building blocks it requires for growth, repair, and disease prevention.

Regular exercise, in addition to a balanced diet, is essential for achieving and maintaining a healthy weight. Physical activity increases caloric expenditure, strengthens muscles, and improves overall health. For overall health, the American Heart Association recommends 150 minutes of moderate-intensity aerobic exercise or 75 minutes of vigorous aerobic exercise per week, as well as strength training exercises at least twice a week.

Brisk walking, cycling, and swimming are examples of moderate-intensity aerobic exercise. Vigorous aerobic exercise can include running, HIIT workouts, or high-intensity cycling. Strength training exercises can include weight lifting, resistance band exercises, or bodyweight exercises like push-ups or squats.

A balanced diet and regular exercise may lower the chance of acquiring chronic illnesses such as heart disease, type 2 diabetes, and some forms of cancer. Additionally, maintaining a healthy weight via food and exercise can enhance quality of life and extend lifespan.

CHAPTER 4

DIET AND NUTRITION

A healthy diet that is balanced and contains a range of nutrient-dense foods may give the body the essential nutrients, vitamins, and minerals needed for optimum health and performance. Consuming a high-calorie diet may have a substantial influence on the prevention and treatment of many chronic health disorders, including obesity, cardiovascular disease, diabetes, and cancer.

A calorie-controlled and nutrient-dense diet is often suggested for weight management, which may involve limiting or eliminating high-calorie, low-nutrient meals and increasing intake of low-calorie, high-nutrient foods such as fruits, vegetables, lean meats, and whole grains. Limiting or eliminating sugary beverages and alcohol may also assist in decreasing calorie consumption and perhaps improve overall health results.

While there is no one-size-fits-all approach to food and nutrition, working with a healthcare professional or registered dietitian to build a plan that is personalized to individual requirements, preferences, and health objectives is crucial. In rare circumstances, nutritional supplements or specialized diets may be advised to treat particular nutrient shortages or health concerns.

A good diet and correct nutrition may have mental health advantages in addition to physical health benefits since poor nutrition has been related to an increased risk of depression, anxiety, and other mental health concerns. A diet rich in fruits, vegetables, whole grains, and lean meats offers the vitamins, minerals, and antioxidants essential to maintain a healthy brain and boost mental wellness.

It is also crucial to remember that cultural and socioeconomic variables might impact an individual's access to and intake of healthy foods. For example, certain areas may have limited access to fresh fruit and whole grains, leading to a dependence on processed and high-calorie diets, which may result in inequities in health outcomes and raise the risk of chronic illnesses.

Making minor modifications, such as introducing more fruits and vegetables into meals or reducing high-calorie snacks, may have a substantial influence on overall health results. Working with a healthcare physician or registered dietitian may give tailored direction and assistance to attain maximum health and well-being via adequate nutrition.

Nutritional Needs for a Healthy Diet

A healthy diet fits an individual's nutritional needs. Nutritional needs relate to the number and kinds of nutrients that a person requires to sustain their body's health and function. These nutrients may be gained from the meals we consume or supplements in times of insufficiency.

Carbohydrates, proteins, lipids, vitamins, minerals, and water are the six groups of vital nutrients. Each of these groups has a distinct role in the body and is essential for proper operation.

carbohydrates are the body's major source of energy and should account for the bulk of your calorie intake, with a concentration on complex carbs such as whole grains, fruits, and vegetables.

Proteins are needed for tissue maintenance and repair, as well as immunological function, and may be found in lean meats, fish, beans, and nuts.

Unsaturated fats found in nuts, seeds, and avocados are considered beneficial fats as they aid with energy production, insulation, and brain function.

Vitamins and minerals are essential for the normal functioning of several biological systems and may be received by eating a variety of fruits, vegetables, and lean meats. Water is necessary for optimum hydration, digestion, and waste removal.

A healthcare professional or qualified dietitian may aid in evaluating individual nutritional requirements and designing a tailored meal plan to fit these demands.

A good diet is vital for general health and the avoidance of chronic diseases such as obesity, heart disease, diabetes, and cancer. Consuming a well-balanced diet rich in a variety of nutrient-dense foods may aid individuals in reaching their nutritional demands.

It is suggested to adopt a diet rich in fruits, vegetables, whole grains, lean proteins, and healthy fats while reducing processed and high-calorie meals, and to drink plenty of water to keep hydrated.

Supplementation may be useful in addition to a well-balanced diet for certain folks who may not get enough nutrients by food alone, such as those with specific nutritional shortfalls or vegans and those who adopt a limited diet or vegetarians. Understanding and managing nutritional requirements is crucial to eating a balanced diet and promoting overall health and well-being.

<u>Macronutrients and Micronutrients</u>

Macronutrients and micronutrients are two kinds of nutrients that are necessary for having a healthy body. Macronutrients comprise carbohydrates, proteins, and fats, while micronutrients include vitamins and minerals. Both macronutrients and micronutrients have a crucial role in supporting health and preventing sickness.

Carbohydrates are the principal source of energy for the body. They are broken down into glucose, which is required by the body for energy. Carbohydrates are found in a variety of foods, including fruits, vegetables, grains, dairy products, and legumes. They are classified as either simple or sophisticated. Simple carbohydrates, such as those found in refined grains and processed foods, are readily broken down and may induce elevations in blood sugar levels. Complex carbohydrates, such as those found in whole grains and vegetables, are broken down more slowly, delivering a longer extended source of energy.

Proteins are required for cell development and repair of tissues in the body. They are composed of amino acids, which are the building blocks of proteins. Proteins are found in a range of meals, including meats, fish, poultry, dairy products, and legumes. There are nine important amino acids that the body cannot generate, and they must be absorbed from the diet.

Fats are a critical source of energy for the body and are essential for the absorption of certain vitamins. They are found in several foods, including oils, nuts, seeds, fish, and meat. Fats are classified into two types: saturated and unsaturated. Saturated fats, which are contained in animal products and some processed foods, may enhance cholesterol levels and increase the risk of heart disease fe. Unsaturated fats, which are found in nuts, seeds, and fatty fish, are considered healthier fats.

In addition to macronutrients, micronutrients are equally crucial for preserving health. Micronutrients comprise vitamins and minerals, which are needed in minute amounts nevertheless are crucial for good physiological function. Vitamins are chemical compounds that are vital for optimal growth and development. Minerals are inorganic compounds that are important for a variety of processes in the body. Both vitamins and minerals are found in a range of foods, including fruits, vegetables, dairy products, and meats.

Macronutrients and micronutrients not only give energy and support physiological functions, but they also play specialized roles in protecting health. For example, carbohydrates are important for cognitive function and physical activity. Proteins are necessary for forming and repairing tissues, generating enzymes and hormones, and sustaining the immune system. Fats are essential for absorbing and distributing fat-soluble vitamins and for managing body temperature.

Micronutrients are also necessary for various functions in the body. For example, vitamin C stimulates the immune system and is necessary for collagen synthesis, which is crucial for skin health. Vitamin D is essential for bone health and immunological function. function. Calcium is vital for bone health and muscle function. Iron is essential for the formation of red blood cells. Deficiencies in either macronutrients or micronutrients may lead to health issues. For example, a diet that is rich in saturated fats and lacking in fiber may elevate the risk of heart disease, while a diet that is low in protein might lead to muscle loss and weakness. Deficiencies in vitamins and minerals may lead to a range of health difficulties, including anemia, decreased immune system, and bone loss.

In addition to the types of nutrients, it's also vital to analyze the quality of the foods that we ingest. Highly processed meals and those with added carbohydrates and fats may give calories but may lack the nutrients that are required for maximum health. Whole, minimally processed meals, such as fruits, vegetables, lean meats, and whole grains, are normally more nutrient-dense and are better for overall health.

Macronutrients and micronutrients serve independent but vital roles in maintaining optimal health. Eating a well-balanced diet that includes a variety of nutrient-dense foods is crucial for sustaining physiological processes and lowering the risk of chronic diseases.

Meal Planning for Weight Loss

Meal planning is an essential component of any weight control regimen. It comprises picking foods and meals that are healthful, calorie-controlled, and tailored to individual needs. Clinically, meal planning for weight loss requires a careful study of the individual's existing eating habits, lifestyle, and health status. From this review, a registered dietitian or healthcare professional may develop a personalized meal plan that takes into account the individual's dietary preferences, cultural background, and medical concerns.

The main objective of meal planning for weight loss is to produce a calorie deficit, which includes taking fewer calories than the body burns over time. This may be done by decreasing portion sizes, selecting lower-calorie and nutrient-dense meals, and increasing physical activity. A calorie deficit of 500-1000 calories per day may lead to a weight loss of 1-2 pounds per week, which is a healthy and sustainable rate.

A well-balanced meal plan for weight loss should comprise a variety of meals from all nutritional groups. This includes lean protein sources such as skinless chicken, fish, eggs, and plant-based proteins like lentils and soy products. Complex carbohydrates like whole grains, fruits, and vegetables should also be included, as they supply vital vitamins, minerals, and fiber. Healthy fats like nuts, seeds, avocado, and olive oil should also be ingested as they may assist in improving sensations of fullness, which helps reduce overeating.

The meal plan should also take into mind any medical difficulties or food allergies a client may have. For example, a person with diabetes may need to limit simple carbohydrates like sugar whereas someone with celiac disease may need to avoid gluten-containing foods. The meal plan should also be constructed to ensure sufficient nutritional intake, including vitamins and minerals, to maintain overall health and prevent any dietary deficits.

To ensure adherence to the meal plan, it should be adaptable and adaptive to varied settings such as dining out, traveling, and social events. A registered dietician may provide counsel on making suitable food choices in these situations and may assist in adjusting the meal plan as necessary to maintain long-term success.

A well-designed meal plan should address these challenges and offer options for lowering cravings and emotional eating. For example, integrating foods that are strong in fiber and protein may aid in keeping you feeling full and content for extended durations, minimizing the probability of overeating. Smart snacking may also help to regulate hunger and cravings, picking healthy and portion-controlled snacks such as fruits, vegetables, and low-fat dairy products.

Another key component of meal planning is meal frequency and timing. Eating more frequently, such as eating small, frequent meals throughout the day, may assist in managing blood sugar levels and reduce reductions in energy and mood. Additionally, consuming breakfast every day has been associated with improved weight management and overall wellness.

It is vital to remember that meal planning for weight loss does not have to be particularly rigorous or boring. There are many good and healthy meal and snack choices to choose from and having a range of foods and flavors may make meal planning more entertaining.

Meal planning for weight loss covers clinical, psychological, and behavioral components. A well-designed meal plan should reflect an individual's health status, interests, and ambitions, while also addressing usual challenges such as overeating, emotional eating, and food cravings. By following a personalized, adaptable, and delightful meal plan, individuals may accomplish sustained weight loss and boost their overall health and well-being.

CHAPTER 5

EXERCISE

Exercise is a physical activity that entails imposing demands on the body's muscular and cardiovascular systems. During exercise, the body must turn stored energy into useful forms, such as glucose and fatty acids, to power the muscles. This process comprises several physiological changes, including increased heart rate and breathing rate, dilation of blood vessels to boost blood flow to the muscles, and the release of hormones, such as adrenaline and cortisol.

Regular exercise is related to several health benefits, including improvements in cardiovascular health, weight management, and mental well-being. These benefits are considered to be associated with the physiological changes that occur during exercise, such as greater insulin sensitivity, increased muscle mass and strength, and lower inflammation.

The intensity, duration, and frequency of exercise may vary its therapeutic benefits. For example, higher-intensity exercise is related to more cardiovascular advantages but may be more challenging to sustain for extended lengths. Additionally, the form of exercise could affect its impact on the body. For example, aerobic exercise, such as running or cycling, benefits cardiovascular health, while strength training boosts muscular growth and strength.

It also has a huge impact on numerous other facets of health. Regular exercise has been demonstrated to promote mental health by decreasing symptoms of anxiety and depression, enhancing mood, and strengthening cognitive function. Exercise may also boost sleep quality, which has major consequences for overall health. Exercise has practical benefits in the treatment of several medical conditions, including cardiovascular disease, diabetes, and obesity. In some instances, exercise may be prescribed as a single therapy, while in others it may be used in combination with other therapies, such as medication or dietary adjustments.

When it comes to establishing an exercise program, there are numerous vital things to consider, such as the individual's fitness level, age, and health status. It's vital to start at a level that is appropriate for the individual and to steadily boost the intensity, duration, and frequency of exercise as their fitness level grows. Additionally, individuals should consider merging a variety of exercise sorts, such as aerobic activity, weight training, and flexibility exercises, to generate a balanced overall workout.

Exercise is an effective therapeutic intervention for improving health and treating medical diseases, with effects that transcend beyond physiological changes. By introducing regular exercise into their lifestyle, individuals may boost their overall health and wellness, while also reducing their probability of getting chronic problems

Very Low-calorie Diets (Vlcds)

Very Low-Calorie Diets (VLCDs) are a sort of dietary intervention that comprises ingesting far fewer calories than the body burns in a day, frequently between 800 and 1200 calories per day. VLCDs are extensively used as a short-term treatment for obesity, generally lasting between 12-16 weeks.

VLCDs are beneficial for weight loss because they induce a significant calorie deficit, prompting the body to rely on stored fat for energy. This results in fast weight loss, with individuals managing to drop anywhere from 3-5 pounds per week. However, VLCDs are not appropriate for everyone, and should only be taken under the advice of a healthcare specialist.

VLCDs may be related to many probable harmful effects, including weariness, nausea, constipation, hair loss, and gallstones. However, consumers need to know that VLCDs should not be used as a substitute for a balanced, healthy diet. Once the VLCD is finished, patients should gradually increase their calorie intake while maintaining a balanced diet and activity routine to prevent quick weight return.

VLCDs are typically applied in patients with a BMI of 30 or higher, or those with a BMI of 27 or higher with obesity-related comorbidities such as diabetes, hypertension, or sleep apnea. The diets usually comprise taking a low number of carbohydrates, fat, and protein, and sometimes include meal alternatives such as smoothies, soups, or bars.

The early weight decrease associated with VLCDs could be encouraging for patients, leading to increased adherence.

VLCDs should only be conducted under the advice of a healthcare specialist, as they may lead to electrolyte imbalances and other metabolic disorders that require monitoring. Patients on VLCDs should also be observed for the development of any acute or chronic illnesses, such as gallstones, gout, and cardiac arrhythmias.

VLCDs may be an effective approach for weight loss in certain persons, but should not be employed as a long-term therapy for obesity. Instead, VLCDs should be utilized as part of a total weight management program that includes dietary modifications, physical activity, and behavioral counseling to help patients build healthy habits and sustained weight loss

PART 3 HEALTHY LIFESTYLE CHOICES

A healthy lifestyle is crucial for optimal physical, mental, and emotional welfare. Making healthy lifestyle choices means adopting behaviors and habits that enhance general health and limit the risk of chronic diseases. These choices include, but are not limited to:

1. Proper and adequate nutrition: Eating a balanced and nutritious meal plays a key role in supporting a healthy lifestyle. This entails consuming foods rich in nutrients such as fruits, vegetables, whole grains, lean protein, and healthy fats while limiting the intake of processed and high-sugar meals.

2. Regular physical exercise: Exercise and physical activity are crucial for maintaining a healthy weight, decreasing chronic disease risk, and increasing mental health. The Centers for Disease Control and Prevention recommended at

least 150 minutes of moderate physical exercise or 75 minutes of intense activity per week.

3. Good sleep habits: Quality sleep is crucial for overall health and well-being. Adults should try for 7-8 hours of sleep per night to support healthy physical and mental function.

4. Avoidance of harmful substances: This includes lowering or eliminating alcohol intake and avoiding tobacco products and other medications that may damage general health.

5. Stress management: Chronic stress may have harmful implications on physical and mental health. Engaging in activities such as deep breathing, mindfulness, and relaxation practices may help decrease stress levels and promote overall well-being.

6. Regular health check-ups: Regular medical check-ups and screenings for chronic conditions such as diabetes, high blood pressure, and cancer may help discover probable health risks early and improve overall health outcomes.

Another vital aspect of a healthy lifestyle is maintaining social connections and relationships. Studies have shown that social support may have a favorable effect on physical and mental health by decreasing stress, boosting mood, and encouraging resilience.

Engaging in activities that increase social relationships, such as volunteering, engaging in clubs or hobbies, or joining a sports team, may have a substantial effect on overall well-being.

Taking care of one's mental health is a critical element of a healthy lifestyle. This may involve strategies such as mindfulness meditation, cognitive-behavioral therapy, and relaxation techniques. These approaches may help lessen anxiety and depression, increase self-esteem, and build resilience.

Another crucial component in sustaining a healthy lifestyle is minimizing exposure to environmental contaminants. This may be done by purchasing organic or pesticide-free meals, using non-toxic household cleaners, and avoiding exposure to smoking, pollution, and other harmful substances.

Adopting healthy lifestyle choices requires making excellent modifications in diet, physical activity, sleep patterns, stress management, and avoiding harmful substances. These practices, together with periodic medical check-ups, may boost overall health and minimize the risk of many chronic disorders.

CHAPTER 6

GROCERY SHOPPING FOR A HEALTHY DIET

Grocery shopping for a healthy diet includes making conscious judgments about the foods and liquids that one consumes. This process begins with planning, as individuals should consider their dietary needs, likes, and finances when choosing meals and beverages. A healthy diet may incorporate a variety of complete foods from numerous nutritional groups, including fruits, vegetables, whole grains, lean meats, and healthy fats.

When food shopping for a healthy diet, it is vital to read labels and pay attention to nutritional information. Foods that are high in sugar, salt, and saturated fats should be avoided or consumed in moderation as they may contribute to chronic health concerns such as obesity, type 2 diabetes, and heart disease. Instead, consumers should prioritize meals and beverages that are lower in added sugars, salt, and saturated fat, while being richer in vitamins, minerals, and fiber.

Another key component of grocery shopping for a healthy diet is preferring fresh, natural foods over processed and packaged items. Fresh fruits and vegetables, lean meats, and whole grains are nutrient-dense and may give the vitamins and minerals essential to preserve optimal health. Processed and packaged meals often include added sugars, salt, and unhealthy fats that may contribute to a variety of health risks.

Planning meals and making a list may also aid customers in grocery shopping for a balanced diet. By making a meal plan and shopping list, people may ensure they have the essential goods and resources on hand to make healthful meals throughout the week. This may also help minimize food waste and save money over time.

Finally, grocery shopping for a balanced diet takes a dedication to picking healthy products. This requires being attentive to the meals and beverages that one consumes and making conscious decisions about what to purchase and consume. By selecting full, nutrient-dense meals and avoiding foods heavy in sugar, salt, and toxic fats, individuals may promote maximum physical and mental health.

Tips for Healthy Grocery Shopping

Grocery shopping for a healthy diet needs a consideration of an individual's nutritional requirements, preferences, and budget. A healthy diet consists of complete foods from many dietary groups, such as fruits, vegetables, whole grains, lean meats, and healthy fats. A balanced diet should be reduced in added sugars, salt, and saturated fat while being richer in vitamins, minerals, and fiber.

Processed and packaged meals often include added sugars, salt, and unhealthy fats that may contribute to a variety of health risks. Therefore, it is vital to favor fresh, full meals over processed and packaged foods. Planning meals and developing a shopping list may also aid in guaranteeing that people have the essential goods and resources on hand to make healthful meals throughout the week.

excellent ideas for healthy food buying.

1. Store the perimeter of the store. The outer edges of grocery stores frequently include fresh veggies, lean meats, and dairy goods. By remaining peripheral, shoppers may avoid many of the highly processed and packaged foods found in the inner aisles.

2. Read food labels carefully. When buying packaged foods, it's vital to examine the nutrition labels to assess the nutritional content. Look for foods that are low in saturated fat, added sugars, and salt, and high in fiber, vitamins, and minerals.

3. Choose lean proteins. Opt for lean meats, such as chicken or fish, and plant-based protein sources like beans and lentils. Avoid foods that are rich in saturated fat and processed meats, such as deli meats and sausages.

4. Buy in quantity. Purchasing greater quantities of healthy basic foods, such as rice, oats, and almonds, may be cost-effective and give meal planning flexibility.

5. Don't shop when hungry. Going grocery shopping on an empty stomach could lead to impulsive purchases of unhealthy snacks and quick meals. Eating a healthful snack before heading to the grocery may help prevent this.

Making healthy choices when grocery shopping needs a commitment. It requires being attentive to the meals and beverages that one consumes and making deliberate decisions about what to purchase and consume. By choosing a balanced, nutrient-dense diet and avoiding foods heavy in sugar, salt, and toxic fats, individuals may promote maximum physical and mental health. A balanced diet may aid in lowering the risk of chronic diseases such as obesity, type 2 diabetes, and heart disease.

Healthy Meals And Snacks

Consuming balanced meals and snacks is crucial for maintaining good health and preventing numerous chronic illnesses. The body requires a spectrum of nutrients such as carbohydrates, proteins, fats, vitamins, and minerals to work efficiently. A balanced diet that includes complete meals from varied food groups may help give these nutrients.

Healthy meals and snacks help regulate blood glucose levels, giving sustainable energy throughout the day. This means that individuals are less prone to endure dips in energy and desire for unhealthy meals high in sugar and harmful fats. A nutritious diet may help aid in keeping a healthy weight, as whole foods tend to be fewer in calories and higher in fiber, enhancing satiety and lowering the likelihood of overeating.

A balanced diet may help prevent chronic diseases such as heart disease, diabetes, and certain kinds of cancers. Consuming a diet that is plentiful in fruits, vegetables, nutritious grains, and lean meats has been connected with a lower risk of chronic diseases. Conversely, eating a diet that is rich in processed and junk foods, high in saturated fats and sugar has been connected to an increased risk of chronic diseases.

Consuming healthful meals and snacks could also have major effects on mental health. Studies have revealed that a balanced diet helps lessen sensations of anxiety and sorrow. This may be connected to the fact that a proper diet may aid in regulating neurotransmitters in the brain that are involved in mood regulation.

Healthy eating habits acquired in infancy may have long-term advantages for health. Children who consume nutrient-rich meals have been observed to have higher scholastic success, improved behavior, and decreased risk of chronic diseases later in life.

However, it is crucial to remember that only swallowing healthy meals is not enough for optimal health. The technique by which meals are made and consumed may also have an influence. For example, deep-frying meals or boiling them at high temperatures may release hazardous compounds, while eating hurriedly or while disturbed could decrease nutrient absorption and increase the risk of gastrointestinal diseases.

Therefore, it is vital to also adopt good cooking and eating habits. This comprises cooking with healthy oils such as olive oil, adopting cooking methods that retain nutrients, and digesting meals carefully and without interruption.

Consumption of nutritious meals and snacks is an essential component of a healthy lifestyle. By prioritizing balanced, nutrient-rich meals and preparing and eating intelligently, individuals may achieve maximum physical and mental health.

CHAPTER 7

CREATING A HEALTHY ENVIRONMENT

Creating and maintaining a healthy environment is a critical factor in promoting good health and preventing chronic diseases. The environment we live in may be characterized in different ways, and it covers both physical and social situations. Physical surroundings could include our homes, workplaces, schools, communities, and even the natural environment. Social environments could include our family, friends, and community.

A healthy environment improves well-being by fostering healthy behaviors and offering access to tools that support great health. By contrast, an unhealthy environment may lead to poor health results, restricted access to resources, and unpleasant social interactions. For example, living in a location with poor air quality boosts the risk of respiratory illness, and living in areas without access to nutritional meals or safe places to exercise may lead to obesity and related disorders.

Creating a healthy environment includes addressing the causes that contribute to adverse health outcomes and supporting resources that promote good health. This includes actions to improve the physical and social environment, such as boosting air quality, providing safe spaces to exercise, and promoting healthy behaviors through education.

To develop a healthy environment, an understanding of the geography of the ecosystem in the problem is vital. For instance, in a workplace, an evaluation of the environment could aid in uncovering probable problems such as harmful working conditions or ergonomic difficulties. Steps may then be taken to lessen these risks and promote better health.

In schools, promoting healthy behaviors may be supported by giving opportunities for physical activity and access to nutritional meals in the school cafeteria. Community-based efforts may also be beneficial, such as providing safe locations to walk or bike, or organizing community events focused on promoting healthy behaviors.

Creating a healthy environment demands collaboration and joint responsibility across many sectors, stakeholders, and levels. Effective interventions must take into account the distinctive needs and interests of various groups, and engage them in suggesting solutions and creating strategies for implementation.

To build and maintain a healthy environment is crucial for maintaining good health and preventing chronic illness. This means addressing the unique challenges that contribute to poor health outcomes and supporting resources that promote good health. Such interventions comprise multiple sectors, stakeholders, and levels working cooperatively to minimize environmental risks, promote healthy behaviors, and deliver resources that support and sustain health and well-being.

<u>Importance of Social Support</u>

The notion of social support refers to the resources and help that come from social networks such as family members, friends, peers, and community groups. Social support has a significant role in the mental and physical well-being of individuals, and evidence reveals that it has a big effect on health outcomes. Social support has been proven to play a critical function in decreasing stress, alleviating depression and anxiety, preventing chronic illness, and boosting general well-being.

Various research has indicated that social support is vital in promoting healthy health. Social support may work as a buffering mechanism against stress, which is a key cause of chronic illnesses such as heart disease, diabetes, and high blood pressure. A solid social support system may assist in minimizing the effects of stress by delivering emotional support, guidance, and material aid that individuals need to deal with their pressures effectively. This sort of support may lessen the anxiety, fear, and dread associated with stressful circumstances, and it may also assist individuals in dealing with illnesses and recovering more efficiently.

Social support also plays a key role in preventing mental sickness and promoting mental well-being. Studies have revealed that a lack of social support has been connected to an increased risk of acquiring depression and anxiety disorders. Those who have an extensive social network or a strong support system are better able to cope with stress, have fewer symptoms of depression, and tend to have a more positive view of life.

Social support may also increase physical health benefits. Individuals with strong social support networks have been observed to have lower occurrences of chronic illnesses such as cardiovascular disease and cancer. Social support may help individuals to adopt healthier behaviors, such as engaging in physical activity or healthy eating, hence minimizing the risk of chronic illnesses and attaining better health outcomes.

There are several means in which social aid may be offered, including emotional help, educational support, and material aid. Emotional support entails supporting someone with comfort, compassion, and understanding in times of adversity or sorrow. Informational support comprises offering individuals appropriate information and advice, such as treatment alternatives or strategies to manage a chronic disease. Tangible aid comprises delivering tangible assistance, such as transportation to medical appointments or preparing meals.

Social support is vital to promoting good health and preventing chronic illness. A comprehensive support system may operate as a buffer against stress, prevent mental illness, foster healthy behaviors and lifestyles, and enhance general well-being. Individuals need to build and maintain strong social networks as part of good health practices, and healthcare organizations should also stress the provision of social support as part of disease prevention efforts.

Overcoming Emotional Eating

Emotional eating is a condition in which individuals eat in response to emotions such as stress, anxiety, boredom, and sadness rather than physiological hunger. This habit is usually linked with overeating, which may lead to weight gain, obesity, and other health difficulties. Overcoming emotional eating is a therapy method that treats the underlying psychological and emotional factors that underlie this behavior. One effective technique is cognitive-behavioral treatment (CBT). for regulating emotional eating. CBT focuses on altering the beliefs, emotions, and actions that contribute to emotional eating. Individuals are taught to understand their triggers for emotional eating and to acquire strategies for coping with these feelings. For example, if stress is a trigger for emotional eating, individuals may gain stress-management skills such as relaxation exercises or meditation.

Another therapeutic method is mindfulness-based therapy. Mindfulness-based treatments teach individuals to be present and aware of their thoughts and emotions without judgment. This strategy may help people understand their This method may assist individuals in comprehending their ideas and feelings that contribute to emotional eating, without reacting to them. Mindful eating may also be practiced, which comprises being aware of the sensations associated with eating, such as the smell, taste, texture, and warmth of food.

Pharmacological treatments, in addition to psychotherapy, are available approaches that have also proved efficacy in treating emotional eating. drugs such as antidepressants, appetite suppressants, and anti-obesity drugs may be used to address the underlying psychological and physiological components that contribute to emotional eating.

Emotional eating is a sophisticated activity that incorporates not only the psychological components but also the physiological and neurological elements. In particular, emotional eating is connected with changes in brain chemistry and hormones, which could further encourage this practice.

One such hormone related to emotional eating is ghrelin, which is known as the "hunger hormone." Ghrelin levels rise when we are hungry and decrease after we eat, but research has shown that emotional stress may enhance ghrelin levels, leading to increased appetite and food consumption. Conversely, another hormone called leptin, which signifies satiety or fullness, has been demonstrated to be lower in those who engage in emotional eating.

The neurochemistry of emotional eating involves the dopamine reward system, which is active when we participate in rewarding activities, including eating. Research has shown that those with emotional eating tendencies exhibited increased activation in the dopamine reward pathway when they see and consume high-calorie products. The perception of pleasure from eating may immediately soothe negative emotions, leading to the reinforcement of emotional eating habits. Overcoming emotional eating is a multifaceted strategy. that covers the biological, psychological, and social elements that contribute to this habit. By taking measures to control hormones, manage stress, and build healthy behaviors, people may break the cycle of emotional eating and have a more balanced relationship with food.

CHAPTER 8

PREVENTION OF OBESITY

Obesity is a serious public health concern affecting millions of people globally. It is a chronic illness marked by an excess deposition of body fat that may lead to several health difficulties, including cardiovascular disease, diabetes, and various cancers. One of the most successful methods to treat this problem is via preventative initiatives that attempt to encourage healthy diet, physical exercise, and lifestyle modifications.

The prevention of obesity encompasses a multi-faceted approach that targets several elements leading to the condition. These variables include genetic, environmental, behavioral, and socioeconomic factors, which may all increase an individual's risk for obesity.

One of the essential approaches to the prevention of obesity is adopting proper eating habits. This entails supporting the consumption of a balanced diet that is rich in fruits, vegetables, whole grains, and lean protein sources. Additionally, customers are urged to minimize their intake of high-calorie, nutrient-poor meals, such as sugary drinks, fast food, and processed snacks.

Regular physical activity is another crucial aspect of obesity prevention. Participation in regular exercise may help individuals maintain a healthy weight by burning calories, growing muscle, and improving overall health. Additionally, exercise may help decrease stress, boost mood, and create a feeling of well-being.

Prevention of obesity also entails addressing environmental factors that contribute to the condition. This entails improving access to nutritious meals through programs such as community gardens, farmers' markets, and healthy food financing programs. Additionally, boosting active transportation, such as walking or bicycling, and establishing safe areas for physical exercise may help promote healthy habits.

Behavioral treatments targeted at developing healthy habits may also play a significant role in preventing obesity.

These therapies could involve counseling, education, and support groups that emphasize improving self-care, mindfulness, and stress reduction skills. Additionally, initiatives that provide prizes for good conduct, such as gym memberships, may aid in pushing individuals to engage in healthy lifestyle modifications.

Finally, addressing socio-economic variables might also help in obesity prevention. These issues include enhancing the availability of inexpensive nutritional meals and safe physical activity venues in low-income communities. Additionally, offering access to economical healthcare may aid folks in managing chronic health conditions that can contribute to obesity.

The prevention of obesity is a difficult and multi-faceted issue that demands a comprehensive approach addressing numerous elements that contribute to the condition. Promoting healthy eating, and frequent physical activity, and addressing environmental, behavioral, and socio-economic determinants may all have a considerable influence on decreasing the prevalence of obesity and improving overall health outcomes.

Preventing general Obesity

Obesity is a complicated disorder that emerges from the interaction of environmental and inherited elements. It is characterized by an accumulation of excess body fat that may lead to several health concerns, including cardiovascular disease, diabetes, and certain kinds of cancer. General obesity refers to the general rise in body fat, whereas abdominal obesity refers to the accumulation of fat primarily in the abdominal region.

Prevention of general obesity comprises lifestyle adjustments that encourage healthy eating, physical exercise, and behavioral changes. A comprehensive approach is necessary, targeting several causes that contribute to the development of obesity.

One of the most effective strategies for reducing general obesity is promoting appropriate eating. This entails having a balanced diet that incorporates plenty of fruits, vegetables, entire grains, and lean protein sources. Diets that are heavy in fat, sugar, and salt, are related to an increase in calorie consumption and weight gain. Dietitians and nutritionists may make suggestions on excellent eating habits, advise portion amounts, and teach nutrition education. Nutrition education may help individuals understand the significance of a balanced diet and how to make sensible food choices.

Physical exercise has been demonstrated to help prevent general obesity. The guidelines are for people to participate in at least 150 minutes of moderate-intensity physical exercise per week. This includes activities such as brisk walking, swimming, cycling, and weight lifting. In addition, physical activity such as weight lifting, strengthens muscles that in turn burn more calories throughout the day. Physical activity also gives numerous other health benefits, such as decreasing the risk of heart disease, increasing mental health, and encouraging enhanced respiratory health.

Behavioral modifications, including adjusting eating patterns and increasing physical activity, are crucial for sustaining healthy body weight, reducing weight, and preventing future weight gain. Participants may successfully lose weight and prevent weight gain with counseling and support services. These programs offer incentives to modify behaviors, identify behavioral triggers, develop targets, and provide feedback toward accomplishing goals.

Environmental improvements may also help general obesity prevention. They may include governmental regulations that encourage healthy behaviors and improved access to healthier foods, such as zoning rules that favor walkable neighborhoods and transportation laws that support active transportation. Many communities have introduced bike-sharing systems that may be used for commuting, conducting errands, and leisure riding.

Finally, socio-economic factors play a crucial impact in the prevention of general obesity. Reducing poverty rates and making healthier food choices more accessible could boost the long-term health of disadvantaged individuals. Additionally, access to cheap healthcare, including preventative therapies, such as regular check-ups, cancer screenings, and chronic disease management, may increase quality of life and minimize health expenses associated with obesity.

Preventing general obesity is a difficult, complete endeavor that includes the combined effort of education, behavior modification, policy formulation, and environmental and socio-economic interventions. To be effective, these interventions should be adapted to the individual requirements of those at risk and must be sustained over time. By working together, public health practitioners, healthcare providers, policymakers, and citizens may help to lower the prevalence of obesity and promote the overall health of communities.

SUMMARY

Obesity is a chronic condition characterized by an excess accumulation of body fat, which may lead to several health complications. To prevent obesity, a multi-faceted approach is needed, addressing multiple components that contribute to the condition, including genetic, environmental, behavioral, and socioeconomic factors. Strategies for obesity prevention include promoting excellent eating habits, frequent physical activity, addressing environmental and socio-economic factors, and behavioral therapies such as counseling, education, and support groups. Reducing the incidence of obesity involves a comprehensive plan to establish a healthier and more supportive environment for individuals to maintain a healthy weight and improve overall health outcomes.

www.ingramcontent.com/pod-product-compliance
Lightning Source LLC
Chambersburg PA
CBHW070818280726
48660CB00016B/2118